CHAIR YOGA

FOR SENIORS

OVER 50

THE ULTIMATE GUIDE TO 5 MINUTES EXERCISE:

FULLY SEATED POSES FOR THE NEXT 30 DAYS, TO IMPROVE YOUR MOBILITY AND FLEXIBILITY

FELIX RICH

TABLE OF CONTENT

INTRODUCTION

Here's to the life-changing adventure that is **"Chair Yoga for Seniors: The Ultimate Guide to 5 Minutes Exercise."** This thorough approach, designed especially for elders looking to improve their flexibility and mobility, delves into the profound synthesis of movement and mindfulness. Get ready to go on a 30-day journey of totally sitting poses that will guarantee not only physical vigor but also a comprehensive embracing of wellness.

The Influence of Chair Yoga: Accepting Well-Being

Chair yoga is a gateway to wellbeing that exists outside of age barriers, not just as an exercise regimen. Consider your body as a well-tuned instrument, with every action representing a note in the wellbeing symphony. Chair yoga is a mild kind of yoga that helps you connect with your body, mind, and soul via fully seated poses. Imagine yourself in the middle of a forward seated pose. Sensate the lengthening of your spine as well as the embrace of flexibility that extends well beyond the mat.

Think of chair yoga as your reliable guide on your journey towards wellbeing. The positions are an invitation to develop a thoughtful awareness of your body's potential, not just a physical one. Imagine the stress leaving your entire body as you extend into a seated twist, not just your back. Chair yoga transforms into a haven where you can embrace the entirety of your well-being one pose at a time.

Why Five Minutes Count: The Science of Brief But Effective Meetings

Let's now investigate the secret that makes 5-minute chair yoga sessions so effective. These brief but deliberate movements have a significant effect on your body and mind, according to science. Think of it as your daily intake of energy. Think about the sitting cat-cow stance; in a matter of minutes, you awaken your spine and energize your whole body. The quality of interaction is more important than the amount of time spent; much like the effects of a tiny cup of strong herbal tea persist long after the final sip.

These few meetings have a cascading effect on your overall health. Imagine the cumulative effects of practicing chair yoga for five minutes every day: a mild adjustment to your posture, increased mobility, and an increased awareness of your body. Throughout your 30-day trip, it's like sowing seeds of vitality that gradually blossom into a garden of well-being.

Getting Ready: Establishing a Cozy Environment for Chair Yoga

Let's set the mood for your transforming chair yoga session before we get into the poses. Your home turns into a canvas for wellbeing. Think of it as an artist setting up their workspace: cozy chair, gentle lighting, maybe a potted plant for a touch of nature. This is about creating a cocoon of comfort and tranquility, not just about looks. Think of it as a caring atmosphere where every position is a paint brush for your overall masterpiece of wellbeing.

Consider your area as a private sanctuary where you may devote all of your attention to your practice. From being merely a piece of furniture, the chair becomes a hallowed place for study. The atmosphere and energy are set as soon as you sit down to improve your chair yoga experience.

We walk you through 30 days of fully seated positions in the pages that follow, with each day revealing a new aspect of your flexibility and mobility. Prepare yourself for a life-changing encounter where the wisdom of five minutes and the simplicity of a chair lead to wellness. Prepare to take on the ultimate guide to chair yoga for seniors, where each posture represents a step towards becoming a more dynamic, flexible, and harmonious version of yourself.

CHAPTER ONE

The Basis of Chair Yoga

As we set the groundwork for our trip into the peaceful realm of chair yoga, where movement and mindfulness converge, we start here. This chapter delves into the essential components that will mold your 30-day investigation of completely sitting poses: every breath is deliberate, and every posture has a specific goal.

Recognising the Fundamentals: Alignment, Posture, and Breath

1. Breath: Chair Yoga's Regular Heartbeat

The breath is the fundamental component of chair yoga; it is a subtle yet potent energy that guides your entire practice. Think of your breathing as the steady pulse of your health. As you sit in a mountain position, take a deep breath and feel your chest expand. Then let the breath and let the tension leave your body. A dance of vitality is created within, with the breath acting as a guide and coordinating with every action.

2. Posture: Positioning Your Body to Promote Health

Posture is a representation of your inner state and goes beyond just your physical posture. Think about the seated warrior posture in chair yoga. Straighten your back, contract your abdominal muscles, and sense the power within. Consider your body as an energy vessel, with each pose serving as a fine-tuning brushstroke on your posture canvas. You can develop poise off the mat in addition to physical power by practicing conscious alignment.

3. Alignment: Every Pose's Original Design

The blueprint that guarantees your body moves in unison is alignment. For instance, when you perform the seated cat-cow stretch, see your spine as a straight line that stretches with each breath. Incorrect alignment can cause pain or reduce a pose's benefits. Think of it like building a house: a solid foundation guarantees that the building will stand tall. Careful alignment is your guide when practicing chair yoga, making sure every position has a purpose.

4. Using Your Chair as a Mat: Maximizing Seated Posing Opportunities

Your chair is more than just a piece of furniture; it's also your yoga mat and a blank canvas waiting to be painted. Chair yoga offers a special chance to experiment with mobility while receiving complete support during seated positions.

5. Mountain Pose in Sitting: Grounding and Elevating

Imagine sitting in the mountain stance, with your spine tall and your feet flat. Your chair turns into a solid foundation that grounds you, much like the ground does. Sense how your body and the chair are connected, keeping you rooted in the here and now. Imagine reaching for the sky as you extend your arms above your head, connecting with a feeling of loftiness and spaciousness.

6. Bending Forward While Seated: Relaxing Tension

In the seated forward bend, the chair allows for a mild stretch. Imagine allowing the chair to assist your travel by folding forward from your hips. This pose releases tension in your hamstrings and spine, making you exhale metaphorically. The chair serves as a dependable ally, providing encouragement and support as you delve further into the stretch.

Keeping It Balanced: Adding Stability to Your Work

In chair yoga, balance—a fundamental principle of yoga—takes center stage. Poses that include sitting provide a special area for developing grace and steadiness.

7. Tree Pose in Seats: Firm Basis

As you sit in tree pose, your spine lengthens and your feet serve as firmly planted roots on the ground. Because the chair offers stability, you can concentrate on the minute details of balance. Think of yourself as a tree that is softly swaying in the wind. This act of balance cultivates a mental equilibrium as well as improved physical stability—a dance between rootedness and flexibility.

8. Sitting Twist: Discovering Balance

Investigate the sitting twist, in which your rotation is supported by the chair. Imagine the accumulated tension in your spine being released as it unwinds like a wrung-out linen. You can twist further without straining because the chair acts as your anchor. Chair yoga's balancing pose improves flexibility and teaches you how to maintain balance through life's ups and downs.

Through our exploration of the complex dance of breath, posture, and alignment, we have laid the groundwork for chair yoga. The chair transforms from a basic seat to a dynamic mat that supports you on your journey. Imagine each fully sitting pose as a step towards improved mobility and flexibility as we go deeper into the 30-day course. It's a journey where every breath and movement is a brushstroke, helping to create a masterpiece of well-being.

CHAPTER TWO

Start of a 30-Day Journey

Welcome to the thrilling beginning of your 30-day Chair Yoga adventure—a 5-minute daily quest for improved flexibility and mobility. Every day opens a new chapter that reveals fully sitting postures that will strengthen your body and improve your overall health.

Day 1–5: Calm Initiations - Easy Pose Techniques to Wake Up Your Body

The seated cat-cow stretch is a great way to start your journey since it gently stretches your spine and sets the tone for the days to come. Imagine the elegant pose as a gentle morning stretch for your entire body, luring it into a conscious state. During these first few days, chair yoga is all about simplicity. You can start with postures like the sitting forward bend and seated mountain to ease yourself into the rhythm.

☐ Day 1: Cat-Cow Stretch While Seated

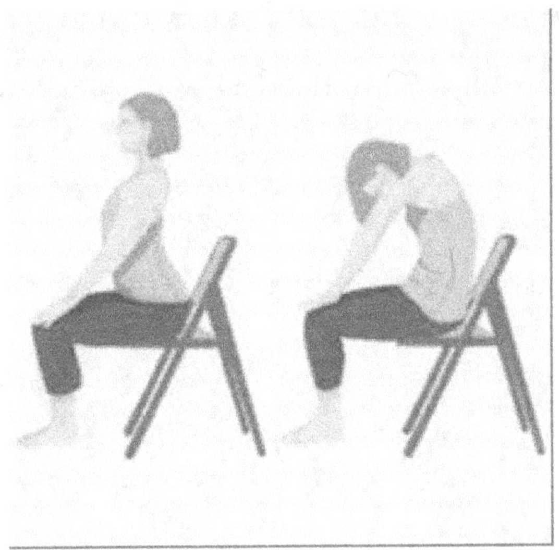

Sit upright, placing your hands just above your knees if you're in a wheelchair, get out of the chair if you can, and set your feet on the floor. If you're using foot pedals, that's okay; you won't be able to stretch your spine as deeply.

Breathe in, bring your head down, bend your knees, and arch your back.

Breathe out, return your hands to the beginning position, raise your head slowly, and straighten your spine.

Repeat three to five times at a slow pace.

☐ Day 2: Mount Everest Pose

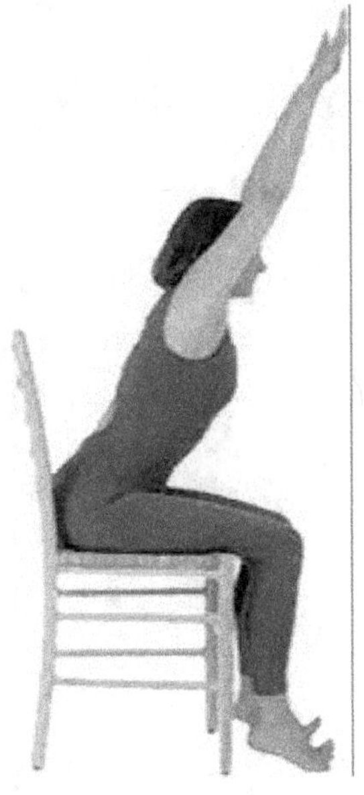

Maintain a straight spine and relaxed shoulders when sitting tall.

Put both of your hands on your knees or thighs.

Breathe in and raise your arms, keeping your palms facing one another.

Breathe out while maintaining your sit bones.

Your spine will lengthen as you feel the strain along your sides.

☐ **Day 3: Forward Bend While Seated**

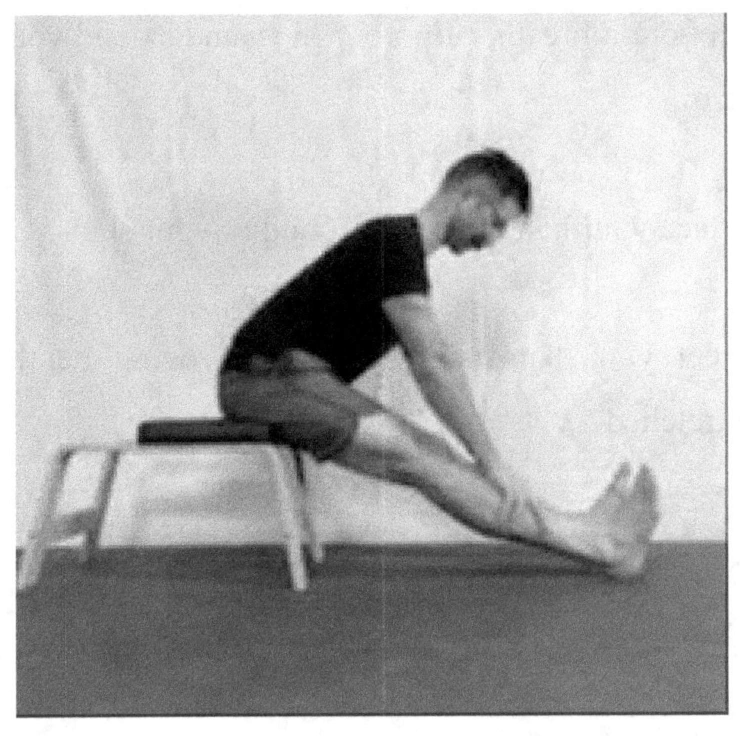

With your feet flat on the ground, take a comfy seat.

Breathe in and extend your back.

Let out a breath, turn your hips, and extend your arm.

Place your hands on the ground or your shins.

Feel your hamstrings and spine being gently stretched.

☐ **Day 4: Stretching while seated**

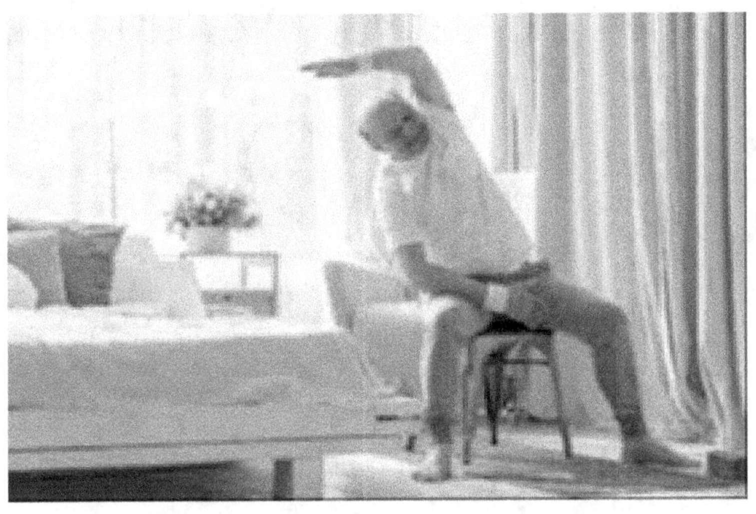

Plant your feet hip-width apart.

Exhale and raise your arms above your head.
Breathe out, slant to one side, and extend your
upper body.

Breathe in and out while holding, experiencing
the elongation.

Breathe in again to the center, then out the other side.

☐ **Day 5: Child's Pose Variation and Seated Relaxation**

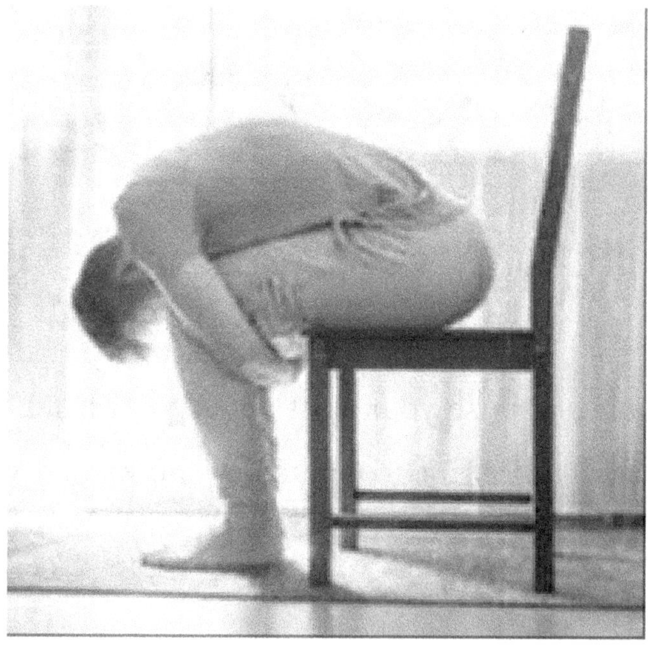

Feet together and knees bowed, take a seat.

Exhale and raise your arms above your head.

Breathe out, turn your hips to face your thighs, and pull your chest in.

Allow your arms to hang or lie flat on the ground.

Feel your lower back gently relax as you take a deep breath.

These easy positions serve as a gentle beginning to chair yoga, awaking your body bit by bit and preparing it for the days to come. As you explore each pose, keep in mind to breathe deeply and pay attention to your body.

Turn your attention to doing seated leg lifts and twists to develop a strong core foundation. Consider the chair to be your exercise equipment, providing resistance as you work your abdominal muscles. Consider the process of strengthening as if you were weaving a shield of defense around your core, which is necessary to keep your balance, stability, and spine supported.

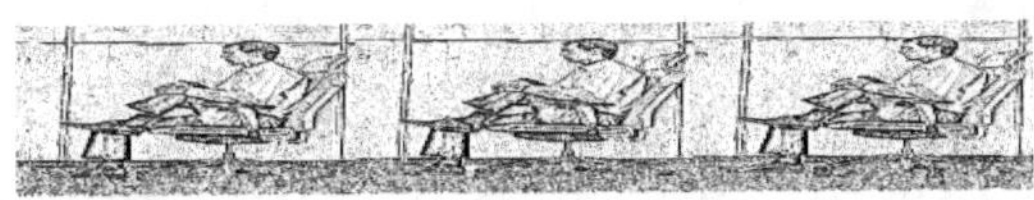

With your feet flat on the ground, sit tall.

Take a breath and extend one leg straight ahead of you.

Breathe out and bring the leg back down.
Continue on the opposite side.

For the movement to be supported, engage your core.

- **7 th Day: Sitting Twists**

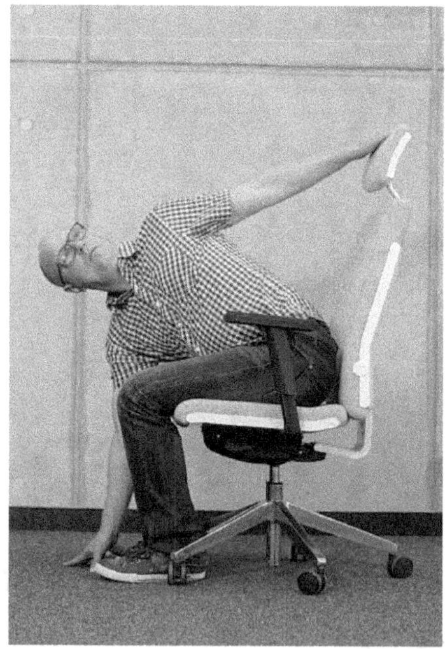

Hands on knees and feet flat on the seat.

Breathe in and extend your back.

Breathe out, turn to the side, and support yourself with your hands.

Breathe in again to the center, then out the other side.

Twisting causes your core to get activated.

- **Day 8: Knee Tucks While Seated**

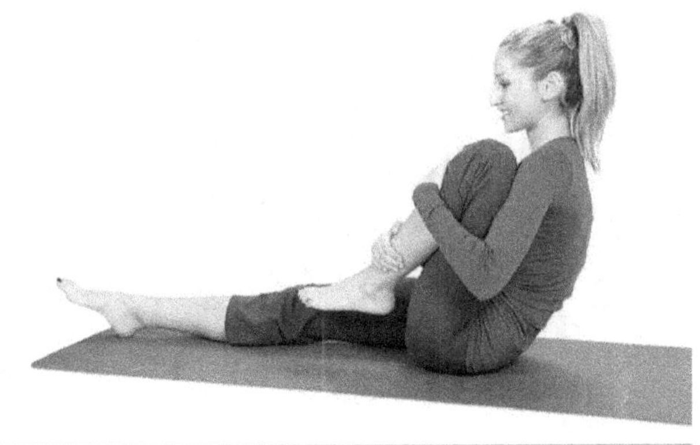

Elevate your feet off the ground when sitting.

As you inhale, pull your legs up to your chest.

Lean back and spread your legs as you exhale.

Throughout, keep your abdominal muscles active.

Feel the core engagement as you repeat this movement.

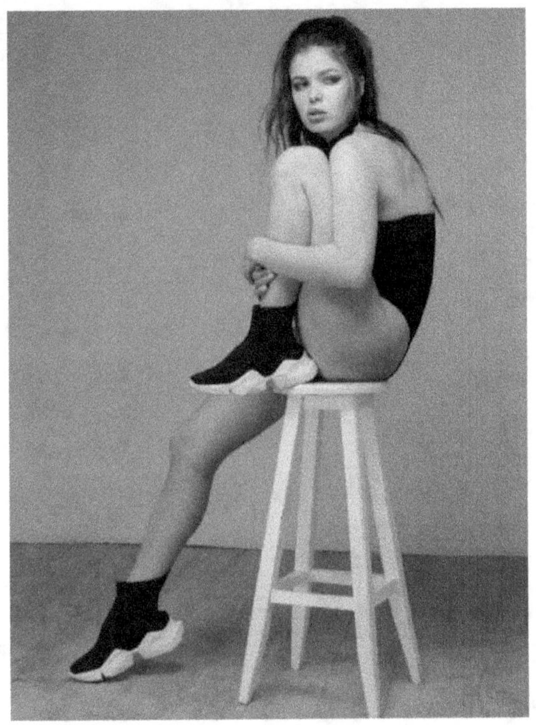

Place your feet together while sitting.

Take a breath and raise a leg to the side.

Breathe out and bring the leg back down.

Continue on the opposite side.

To raise the leg, concentrate on engaging your core.

- **Day 10: Crunches on a seated bicycle**

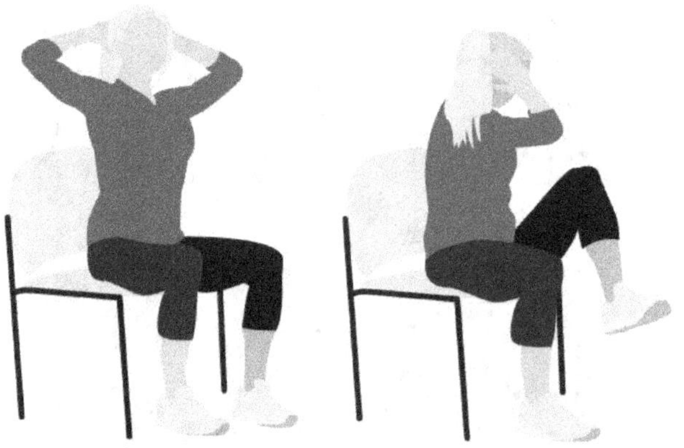

Place your hands behind your head as you sit.

Taking a breath, lift one leg to your chest.

Twisting to move the opposing elbow towards the knee, release the breath.

Return your breath to the center and swap sides.

When you complete these bicycle crunches, notice how your core rotates.

You may support your general well-being by developing stability and strength at the center of your body with the aid of these seated core-strengthening poses. Pay attention to your body during any exercise, and modify the intensity as necessary.

Take on side stretches and seated forward bends to progressively increase your flexibility. Envision these positions as the keys to a more flexible version of yourself. For example, the seated side stretch promotes better torso flexibility by gradually opening your rib cage. The growth of each day builds on the previous one, gradually and mindfully pushing your boundaries.

1. Day 11: Bending Forward and Reaching

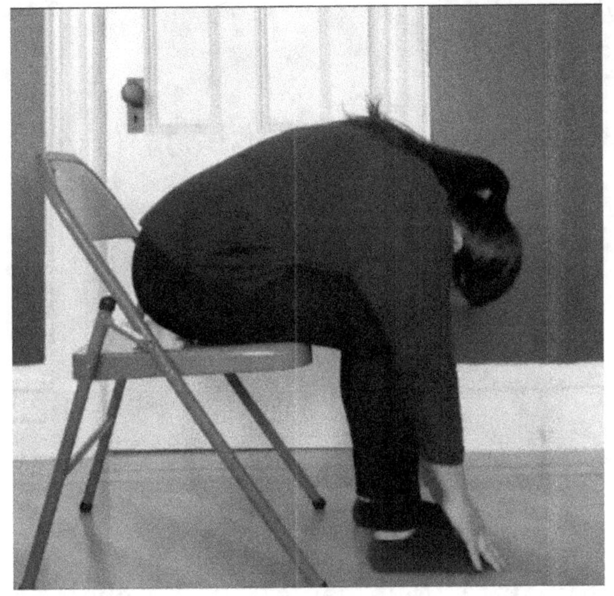

Choose a chair that is steady and won't tip over, and place it away from the desk.

Position yourself close to the chair's edge, keeping your feet firmly planted on the ground and spaced 6 to 10 inches (25.4 cm) apart.

Till the chest makes contact with the thighs, slowly bend forward.

Allow the head to naturally droop. Let the arms dangle at your sides. Shut your eyes.

Breathe deeply and allow gravity to extend your back. Feel all of your shoulder tension release. Take two minutes to relax in this position.

To rise, place your hands on the chair's sides, press down, and raise your torso while taking a breath. After straightening up, breathe twice slowly before going back to the day's activities.

2. Day 12: Extended Arm Variation - Seated Side Stretch

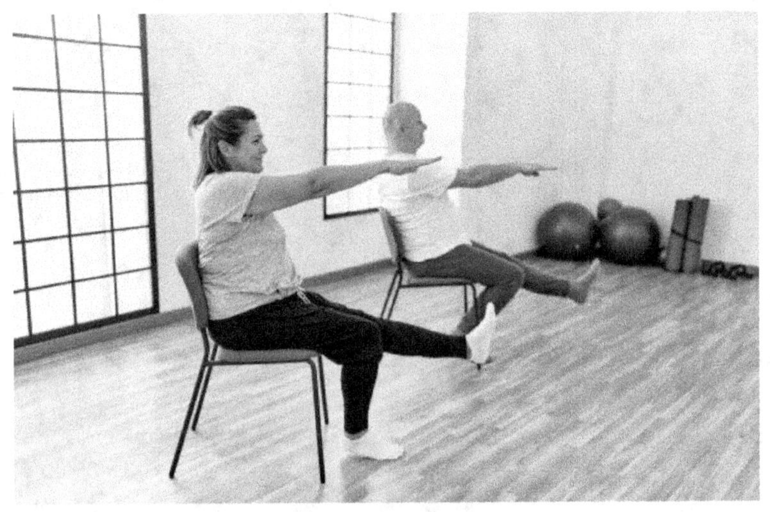

Sit with your legs out in front of you.

Breathe in, extend one arm above you.

Breathe out and sag slightly to the side.

Sensate the strain on your body's side.

Breathe in again to the center, then out the other side.

3. Day 13: Forward Bend While Sitting Wide-Legged

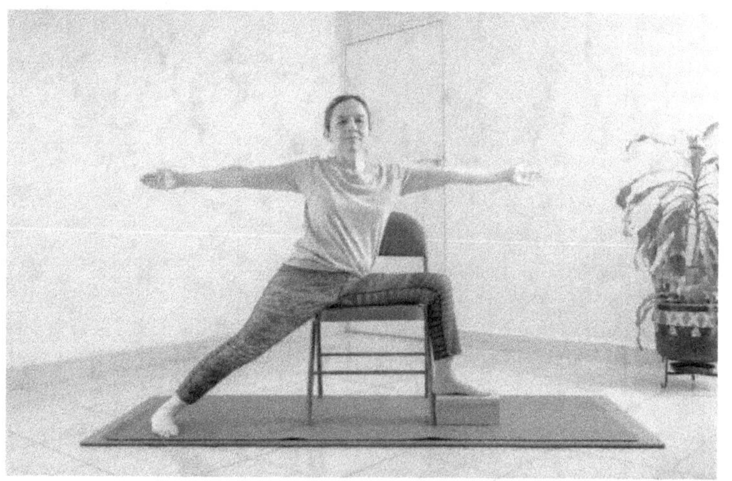

Sit with your legs wide apart.

Breathe in and extend your back.

Let out a breath, bend at the hips, and extend your arm.

When you fold, maintain a straight back.

Sensate the strain in your groin and inner thighs.

4. Day 14: Extended Leg Variation - Seated Twist

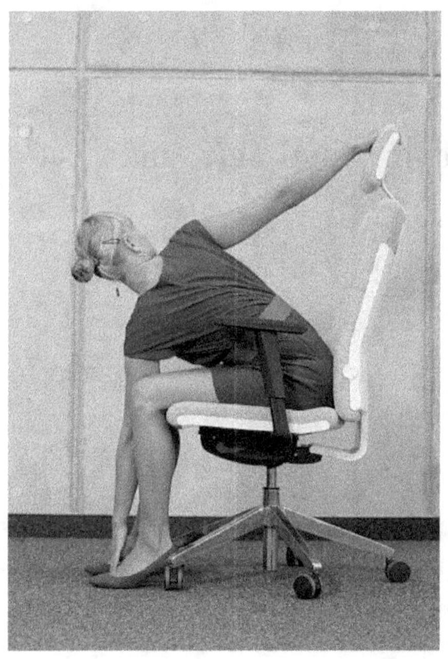

Lean one leg forward and the other bent while seated.

Breathe in and extend your back.

Let go and turn to face the outstretched leg.

To further intensify the twist, use your opposing arm.

Stretch along your side and feel your spine rotate.

5. Day 15: Forward Bend with Seated Leg Cross

Cross your legs and sit.

Breathe in and extend your back.

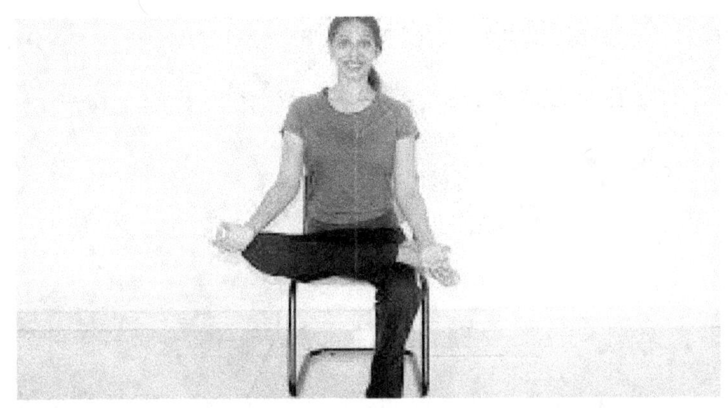

Let out a breath, bend at the hips, and extend your arm.

Let your hands drop to the ground.

Your hamstrings, lower back, and hips should all feel stretched.

The goal of these sitting poses is to progressively increase your flexibility so that your body can adjust and advance. Move carefully as always, and enjoy the feelings that come with each stretch. Pay attention to your body and adjust the poses to what is comfortable for you.

About halfway through your practice, settle into positions of relaxation that are seated. Imagine that the child in the seated position is releasing pent-up tension by surrendering. This is the time to take care of your body, give it a break from more strenuous poses, and let it assimilate the advantages of the preceding days. As you relax and rejuvenate, your chair turns into a paradise.

> **Day 16: Shoulder rolls while seated**

Put your hands on your knees and take a comfortable seat.

As you take a breath, raise your shoulders to
your ears.

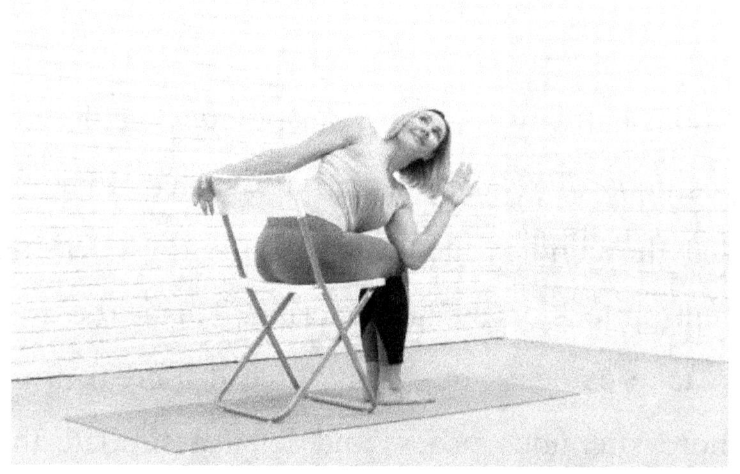

Roll them back and down as you exhale.

As you release the tension in your shoulders,
repeat this movement.

Savor the smoothness of the shoulder rolls,
which encourage calm.

➤ Day 17: Neck stretches while seated

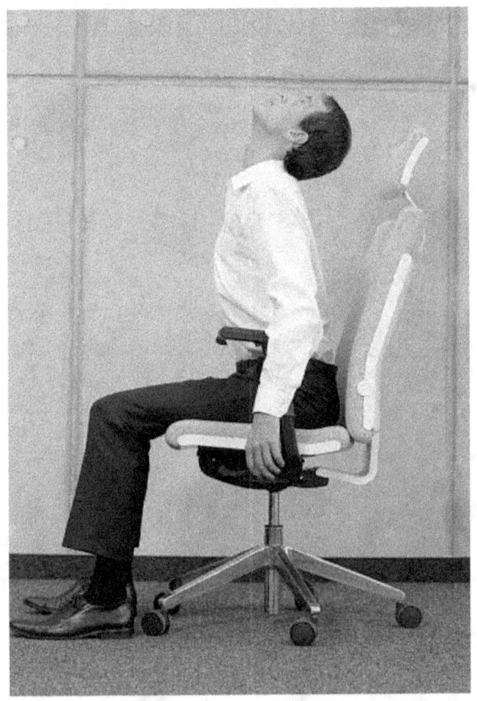

Sit upright in your chair.

Breathe in and extend your neck.

Breathe out, tilt your head to the side, and get a mild stretch.

Breathe in again towards the center and out the other side.

Repeat while releasing the tension in your shoulders and neck.

> ## Day 18: Bending Sideways and Doing a Light Stretch

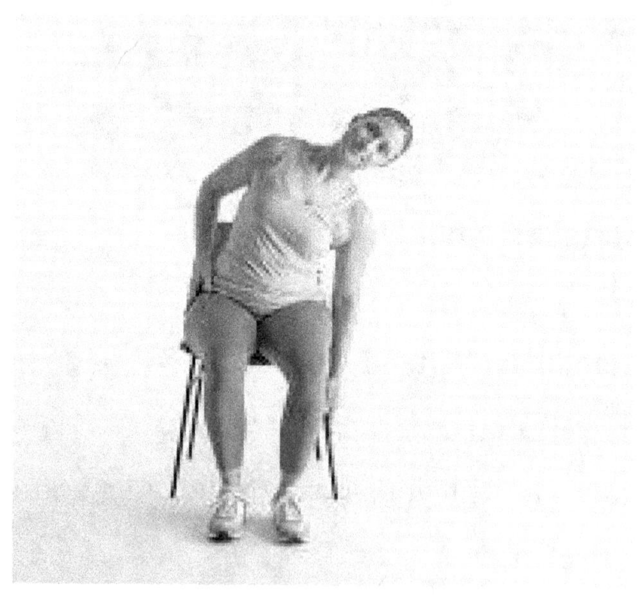

Plant your feet flat on the ground.

Take a breath and raise one arm above your head.

Breathe out and sag slightly to the side.

Sensate the strain on your side.

Breathe in again to the center, then out the other side.

> ➤ Day 19: Opener of the Chest Sitting

Place your hands behind your back and sit up straight.

Squeeze your shoulder blades together as you inhale and open your chest.

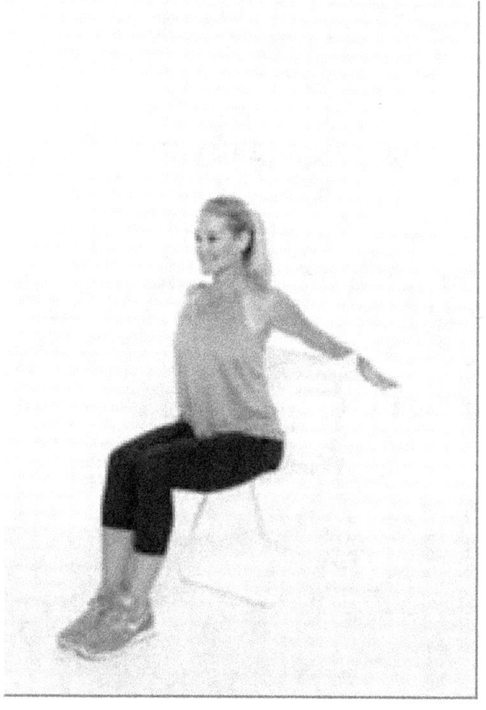

Breathe out, let go, and unwind.

Your chest will expand and tension will release.

To the extent that you feel comfortable, repeat.

➢ **Day 20: Extended Breaths and Seated Relaxation**

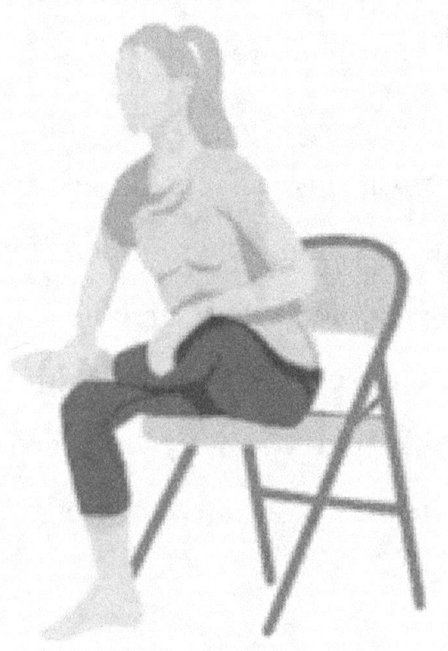

With your feet flat on the ground and hands on your tummy, take a tall stance in your chair.

With your eyes closed, inhale deeply through your nose, sense your hands separating from your body, and exhale through your mouth.

Breathe deeply three times, concentrating on letting your body relax.

These positions for relaxation are meant to assist you in calming down, releasing tension, and relaxing while seated. Breathe your way through each exercise to establish a calm space inside of yourself. Take the poses as far as comfortable and relish the restorative powers of sitting still.

Discover how breath and movement work together in sequences that smoothly transition from one stance to the next. Imagine the sun salutation while seated; it's a flowing sequence that synchronizes breath and movement to create a vibrant dance that happens inside your chair. Your practice is elevated by this confluence, which makes it a vibrant, harmonious experience.

Day 21: Sun Salutation while seated

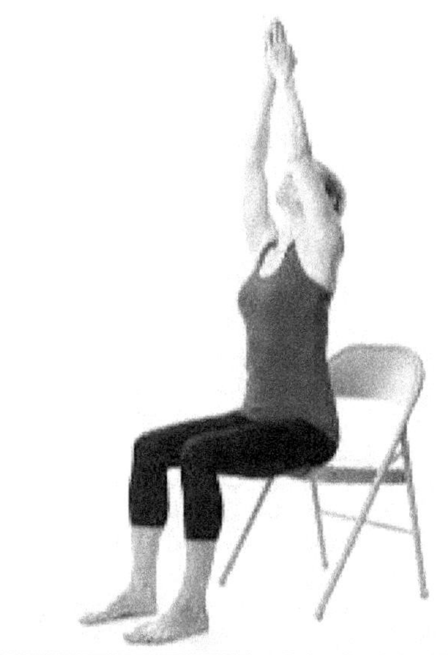

Breathe deeply, raise your arms to the sky, and sit erect.

Let out a breath, turn your hips, and lower your hands.

Exhale and raise your arms once more.

Continue in this manner, matching your movements and breaths.

Breathe and position in a harmonious dance as you feel the flow.

Day 22: The Warrior's Seated Breath

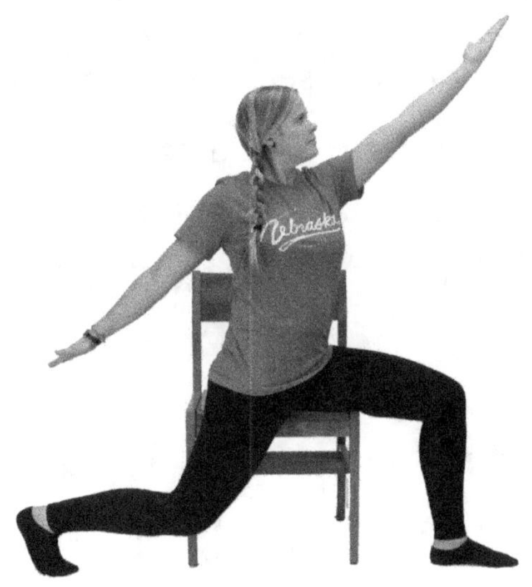

Put your hands on your knees and sit with a tall
spine.

Breathe in and extend one arm, palm up.
Breathe out and bring your hand back to your
side.

Continue on the opposite side.

To create a flowing sensation, synchronize this
movement with your breathing.

Day 23: Cat-Cow Flow While Seated

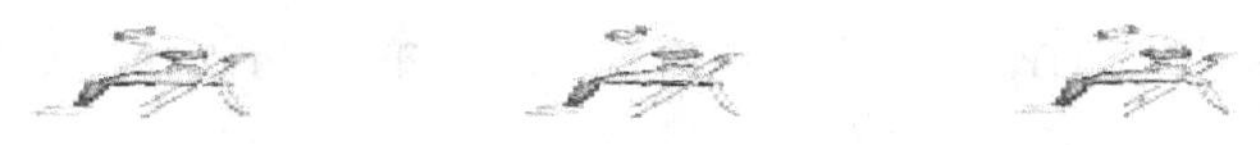

Put your hands on your knees and sit.

Take a breath, raise your chest, and arch your back (Cow).

Breathe out, arch your back, and lift your chin up to your chest (Cat).

Breathe and move together as you perform these motions.

Sensate the soft waves that provide the impression of mobility.

Day 24: Twist Flow While Seated

Hands on knees, sit erect.

Breathe in and extend your back.

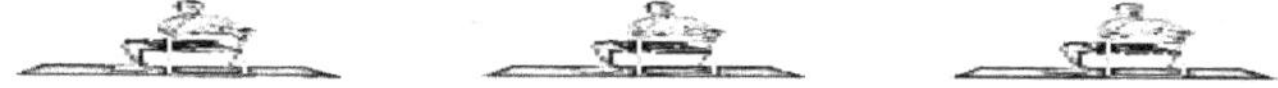

Let go and sway to one side.

Breathe in again towards the center and out the other side.

Breathe your way through each twist, letting your body speak for you.

Day 25: Tree Pose in a Seated Position

Plant your feet flat on the ground.

Exhale, raise one foot, and plant it on the inner thigh of the other person.

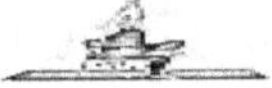 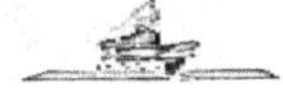 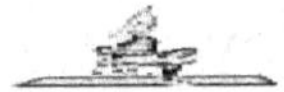

Breathe out and place the foot back down. Continue on the opposite side.

Breathe in a rhythmic and balanced manner as you move through the pose.

Within the confines of your chair, these seated poses create a sense of harmony and flow by combining breath and movement. Accept the way your breath and the poses are related, letting each sequence develop with grace and purpose. Enjoy the harmonic synthesis of chair yoga and change the pace to fit your comfort level.

As the end of your 30-day chair yoga journey draws near, acknowledge and appreciate your accomplishments. Envision yourself becoming proficient in the sitting warrior stance; centered, powerful, and totally present. Recognise the advancements in flexibility and mobility. This stage is about anticipating and reflecting, realizing that chair yoga is a journey rather than a goal.

Day 26: Warriors Pose in Sitting

Place your feet firmly on the floor.

Exhale and raise your arms above your head.

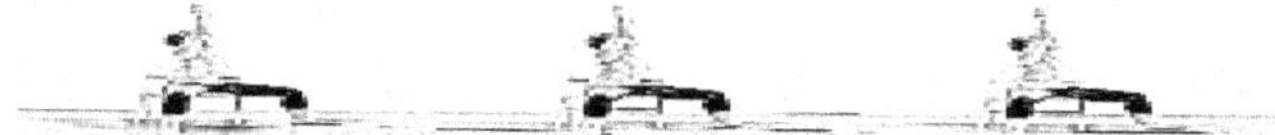

After you release the breath, raise your hands in prayer.

Celebrate your progress and feel centered and strong.

Day 27: Altering the Seated Boat Pose

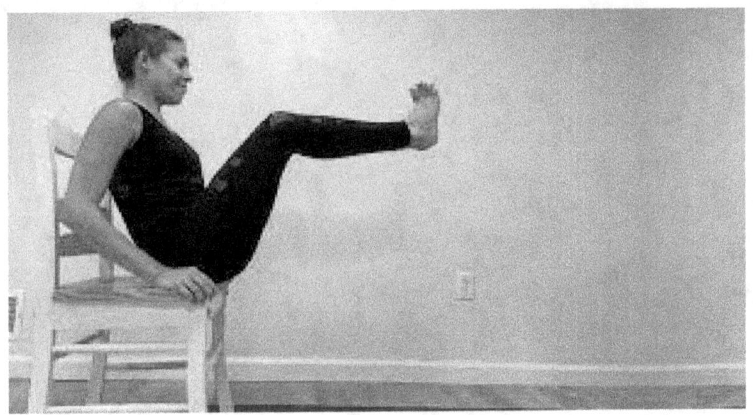

With your feet flat on the floor and your knees bent, sit tall.

Breathe in, raise your legs, and form a 'V' with them.

Let go and contract your abdomen.

Honor the inner power you possess and look forward to what lies ahead.

Day 28: Figure 4 Stretch - Seated Hip Opener

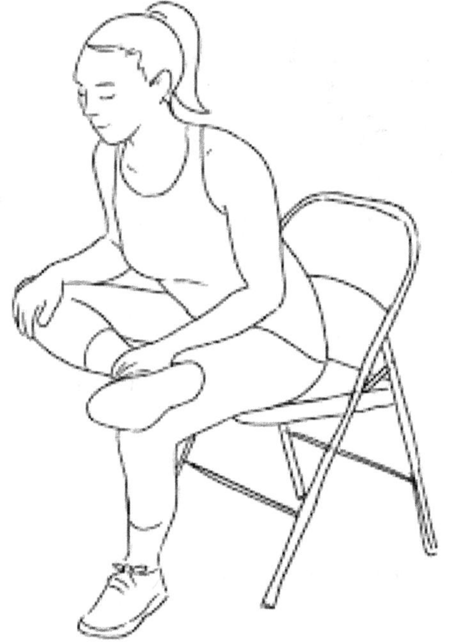

Place your feet flat while sitting.

Place one ankle over the knee of the other.

Breathe in and extend your back.

Breathe out, then softly press your crossed knee.

Enjoy the opening of your hips as a sign of increased flexibility.

Day 29: Heart Opener While Seated

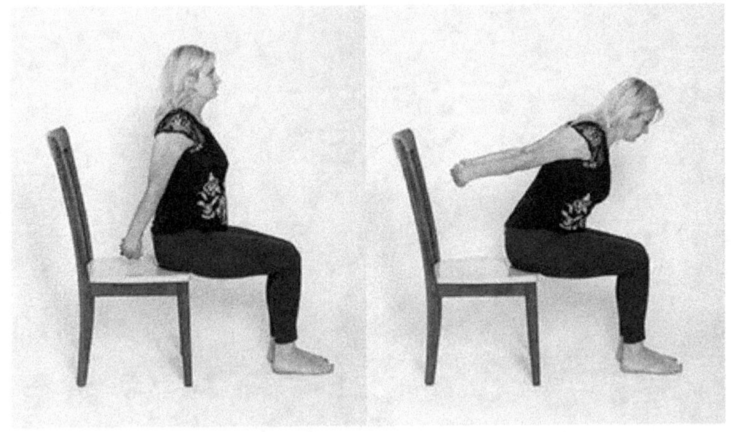

Place your hands behind your back while sitting on the front edge of your chair.

Raise your hands off your back and gently lift your chin off your chest as you take a breath. Lower your hands as you release the breath.

At least twice through, repeat this motion with your breaths. Repeat with a different hand grip.

Day 30: Posing in Victory

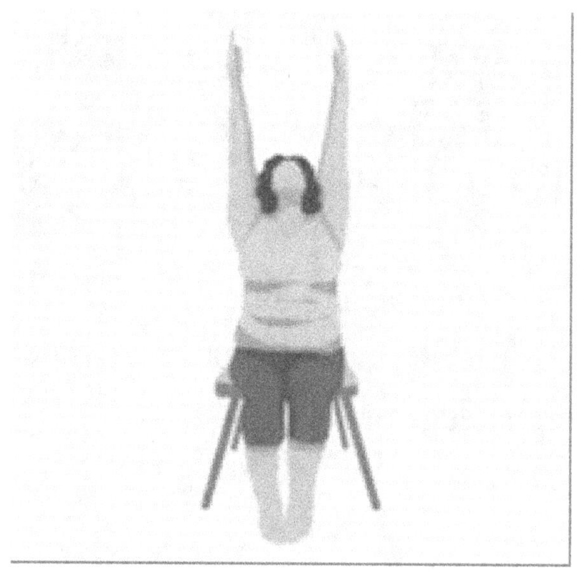

Sit with your shoulders back and relaxed.

Exhale and raise your arms above your head.

Let out a breath and raise your palms in a triumphant gesture.

As you commemorate the end of your 30-day adventure, look forward to more advancements in the future.

As you work your way through these positions, pause to consider your accomplishments over the last thirty days. Recognise the improvements you have experienced in your body, mind, and soul. Celebrate your mastery of these poses and envision a day when practicing chair yoga becomes a lifetime endeavor that promotes growth and well-being.

During these thirty days, your chair becomes a transformational tool that leads you through a variety of fully sat postures. Accept every day as a special chance to improve your wellbeing. The journey's cumulative effect—a tapestry of mobility, flexibility, and a revitalized sense of vitality—is more important than any one position. As you celebrate your successes and look forward to more advancements in the future, get ready to reveal your inner mastery.

CHAPTER THREE

Changing Positions to Fit

Every Body

When it comes to Chair Yoga, inclusion is king. This chapter delves into the skill of customizing poses to meet the demands of each individual, enabling anyone to practice regardless of age or degree of fitness.

Chair Adjustments: Customizing Pose to Meet Needs

- **Warrior Pose in Sitting: Adjusting for Stability**

Start in the seated warrior position, which is a basic stance. If you're looking for support, put a cushion underneath your seat to provide a stable base. With this modification, people who struggle with balance can safely participate in the posture and gain strength without sacrificing safety.

- **Bending Forward While Seated: A Calm Approach**

Take the seated forward bend, a pose that stretches the lower back and hamstrings. A small bend in the knees reduces the amount of tension on the lower back and opens up the posture for people with limited flexibility. This adjustment makes sure that everyone can benefit from the forward bend's revitalizing effects, regardless of flexibility.

Overcoming Limitations: An Elderly Person's Guide to Safe and Effective Chair Yoga

★ Seated Twist that's Friendly to Arthritis: Gentle Relief

The sitting twist can offer mild alleviation to people with arthritis or other joint pain. People can reap the benefits of the twist without aggravating their joint pain by implementing a gradual and controlled movement. Joint health is prioritized in a safe and efficient manner using this method.

★ Assisted Mountain Pose: Increasing Comfort

It might be difficult for seniors to sit still for prolonged periods of time. Introduce the supported seated mountain pose with your hips supported by a folded blanket or cushion. With this adjustment, people can participate in the posture more easily and comfortably while concentrating on their alignment and breathing.

Using Props and Accessories to Enhance Your Poses

> **Enhanced Stretch with Prop Support for Seated Twist**

Props are useful allies that enhance the practice of chair yoga. A tiny pillow between the back and the chair provides a layer of support during a sitting twist, enhancing the stretch in a regulated way.

This improvement guarantees a more profound twist without putting undue strain on the spine, hence enhancing safety and efficacy.

➤ Strap-equipped Chair Yoga Fusion: Fostering Connection and Flow

Incorporate the usage of yoga straps to create a fluid combination of breathing and movement. A strap helps create a smooth transition between positions and connects the arms in poses like the sitting sun salutation. This prop-driven method promotes a conscious connection between movement and breath in addition to improving flow.

When it comes to Chair Yoga for Seniors, flexibility is essential. Everybody can experience the transforming power of completely seated postures, whether they are modified for stability, physical limits are overcome, or the practice is enhanced with props. Let this guide serve as a testament to the adaptability and inclusivity of Chair Yoga—a practice that is praised for its accessibility and suitable for all body types—as we move through the upcoming 30 days.

CHAPTER FOUR

The Relationship Between the Mind and Body

Chair Yoga for Seniors is a colorful tapestry where the body and mind dance in harmony, leading to a 30-day voyage of self-discovery. This chapter explores the deep relationship between the mind and body and shows how Chair Yoga is a transforming practice that goes beyond physical fitness.

Moving Meditation: Chair Yoga as a Conscious Exercise

→ **Mountain Pose in Sitting: Grounding the Thought**

Start your practice with the mountain pose, which is a basic posture that captures the essence of meditation in motion. Imagine yourself as a great mountain, rooted and immovable, as you sit tall. Embrace the calmness of the position and let it be a time for meditation in which the mind finds peace in the simplicity of sitting alignment.

→ Breathing Into It: A Moving Meditation

Make your way to the sitting sun salutation, when each pose transforms into a fluid meditation. Breathe in harmony with the movement of your arms as they rise and fall, creating a dance with your breath. Imagine the sun salutation as a form of movement meditation, with each pose flowing into the next, developing an awareness of the present moment that goes beyond the physical aspects of the practice.

❖ Awareness of Breath in Seated Forward Bend

Turn your attention inward to the breath, which can be a guiding principle when facing obstacles, as you begin the sitting forward bend. Take a deep breath, allowing your chest to expand, then release it as you give yourself up to the forward fold. Your breathing becomes your partner, guiding you through the stretch's feelings with grace and awareness.

❖ Breathing Control in Tree Pose

Accept the subtle interplay of balance and breath that is the seated tree position. Exhale to achieve stability and inhale as you raise one foot to rest on the opposing inner thigh. Imagine that the anchor that keeps you anchored in the here and now is your breath. Beyond the actual task of balancing, each inhale and exhalation becomes a rhythmic representation of equilibrium.

With each pose serving as both an exercise and a conscious investigation, Chair Yoga for Seniors serves as a conduit for the mind-body connection. Over the course of the following thirty days, let your breath to direct your movements, weaving a mindfulness tapestry that enhances the physical advantages of fully seated positions. In Chair Yoga, the body and mind, which are inextricably linked, come together in a dance that transcends the chair, breaks through barriers, and promotes overall wellbeing.

CHAPTER FIVE

Acknowledging the Advantages

Chair Yoga for Seniors shines as a beacon of accessibility and vibrancy in the pursuit of enhanced well-being. This chapter explores the practical advantages, showing how, in just five minutes, fully seated poses may integrate flexibility and mobility into everyday life.

Flexibility Off the Mat: The Benefits of Chair Yoga for Everyday Living

★ Bending Forward While Doing Daily Tasks

The forward-leaning chair becomes more than just a yoga pose. It opens doors to better everyday functioning. Imagine reaching for things on a low shelf or fastening your shoes with ease. This pose helps you become more flexible off the mat as well, which will help you do daily duties with ease and comfort.

★ Increased Shoulder Mobility: Essential for Self-Sufficiency

Imagine the effect on your shoulder mobility as we examine seated shoulder stretches. Reaching is now natural, whether it's picking up a beloved book from a shelf or putting on a jacket with ease. Chair Yoga helps people keep their independence by improving the movement required for daily tasks.

Enhancing Range of Motion for Active Aging: Mobility Is Critical

❖ **Leg Lifts While Seated: Promoting Joint Health**

Including seated leg lifts in your regimen is an investment in joint health as well as fitness. Imagine yourself lifting your legs with a fluidity of movement that helps to strengthen your knees and hips. This increased range of motion demonstrates how effective chair yoga is at maintaining and enhancing joint health for active aging.

❖ **Twist While Seated for Spinal Health**

One of the foundational poses, the seated twist, becomes a protector of spinal health. Imagine the benefits of slowly rotating your spine as you imagine easier turns when driving, reaching for things in the back seat, or comfortably glancing over your shoulder. Chair Yoga becomes an effective technique for preserving the flexibility and agility of the spine.

Chair Yoga: A Painless Solution for Aches and aches

➢ Cat-Cow Stretch While Seated: Relieving Back Pain

For people who have occasionally had back pain, the seated cat-cow stretch proves to be a calming solution. Breathe in as you arch your back and out as you round it; this repetitive movement nourishes and soothes your spine. The soft swaying turns into a healing technique, providing alleviation from the pains associated with a sedentary way of life.

➤ Comfort in Sitting Relaxation Positions

Like the child's pose variation, seated relaxation poses turn into comfort zones. Imagine the peace that will arise as you settle into the posture, relieving stress and giving your tired muscles a break. The tensions and pressures of everyday life are countered by these peaceful Chair Yoga moments.

Let every posture in Chair Yoga for Seniors over the course of the next 30 days be a step towards a life of increased mobility, increased flexibility, and discomfort-free living. The effects are profound and life-changing; they don't stop at the mat; they permeate every aspect of your everyday life.

CHAPTER SIX

Including Chair Yoga in Your Daily Practice

Taking up Chair Yoga for Seniors is a commitment to improve your well-being rather than just an exercise regimen. This chapter delves into the skill of incorporating completely seated postures into your everyday routine, allowing Chair Yoga to become an essential part of your way of life.

Creating a Chair Yoga Routine: Selecting the Ideal Time for You

☐ Morning Booster: A New Beginning

Chair yoga is a great way to start the day because it may energize your body and create a pleasant vibe. Start the day with a strong and resilient mental image of yourself as you sit in the mountain stance. This morning routine prepares your mind for the difficulties and rewards that lie ahead while also improving flexibility.

☐ Afternoon Revitalization: A Midday Energy Boost

Relax and rejuvenate yourself with a chair yoga break in the middle of the day. Easy twists and stretches while seated help release tension that has accumulated over the day. Imagine the side stretch in a seated position as a refreshing break that provides a little period of peace before returning to your duties.

☐ Evening Wind Down: Unwinding for a Sound Sleep

Chair yoga is a great way to end the day and prepare for a restful sleep. Relaxation positions that are done while seated, like the prolonged breath exercise, develop into rituals of peace that set your body and mind up for restful sleep. Accept the evening relaxation as a necessary part of your nightly routine.

Easy Strategies for Maintaining Consistency: Overcoming Typical Obstacles

- **The Benefits of 5-Minute Meetings**

The simplicity of Chair Yoga is one of its greatest qualities. Accept the 5-minute sessions as your go-to tool for maintaining consistency. Finding just five minutes to practice fully seated poses is not only doable, but transformative, even on hectic days. Imagine the effect of all of these quick sessions added together over the course of the following thirty days, progressively improving your mobility and flexibility.

- **Establishing a Specific Area**

Create a special Chair Yoga area in a corner of your living room. Arrange your chair, a cushion, and maybe a little plant to make a calm space. It's easier to include Chair Yoga into your routine and to instill a sense of dedication when you have a dedicated location.

Spreading the Joy: Inspiring Others to Take Up Chair Yoga With You

- **Chair Yoga Get-togethers: A Social Event**

By inviting friends or family to join you in your practice, you can spread the joy of chair yoga. Organize a weekly Chair Yoga meet-up so that people can learn from each other, support one another, and enjoy the advantages of practicing totally sitting positions. Making Chair Yoga a group activity increases its benefits and promotes a feeling of community well-being.

- **Online Link: Online Chair Yoga Classes**

Host virtual Chair Yoga sessions to overcome geographical borders in this digital age. To communicate with friends or relatives who may be located far away, use video conferencing services. As you lead them through poses and share your Chair Yoga experience, you may all enjoy the benefits of increased flexibility and mobility.

Let Chair Yoga transform into a daily ritual of vitality and self-care as you include it into your routine, beyond just a workout. Chair Yoga becomes a lifestyle when you create a schedule, practice consistently, and spread happiness to others. This guarantees that Chair Yoga will continue to improve your health and well-being.

CONCLUSION

As we come to an end of our life-changing Chair Yoga for Seniors experience, take a moment to consider the incredible 30-day journey you have just undertaken. The five minutes it takes to complete each fully seated position has caused a significant change in your range of motion and flexibility. Let's pause to acknowledge your accomplishments and discuss how Chair Yoga can develop into a lifelong wellness practice.

Considering Your 30-Day Metamorphosis

1. Honoring Significant Occasions: From Day 1 to Day 30

Remember back to Day 1, when a path of self-discovery was laid out with gentle beginnings. Every day has been a stepping stone that builds upon the previous one, from the fundamental seated poses to the complex flows. Savor the achievements: when a stretch started to feel more natural, a pose started to flow more naturally, and your breathing naturally matched your movements.

2. Physical Evolution: An Adaptable Tapestry

Think about how your physical health has changed throughout time. The forward bend in your seat that used to feel like a stretch now becomes a natural part of your day. The soft turns that at first needed focus have sunk in as an organic part of your movement vocabulary. Imagine the tapestry of flexibility that these 30 days have woven through them—a tribute to Chair Yoga's transforming potential.

3. Developing Mindful Awareness: Using Breath

Think back on the conscious awareness that was developed over this journey, rather than just the physical gains. The breath has evolved from being merely a soundtrack to movement to a guiding principle. The practice transforms into a moving meditation as you learn to synchronize your breath with positions and breathe through obstacles. This elevated consciousness carries over off the mat and infuses your everyday existence with a sense of serenity and balance.

Senior Chair Yoga: A Lifetime Habit for Health and Well-Being

I. Including Chair Yoga in Your Everyday Routine

As the 30-day programme comes to an end, Chair Yoga is not limited to the contents of this book. Think about how you may adapt these completely sitting positions to your everyday routine. Chair Yoga can be your lifetime partner on your path to well-being, whether you use it for an evening wind-down, a morning ritual, or a midday break.

II. Changing and Growing: Fulfilling Your Changing Requirements

Your body is dynamic, just as life itself. Chair yoga is a dynamic practice that changes to meet your needs as they arise. Chair Yoga develops along with you, whether you're taking on new difficulties, experimenting with different position variants, or going deeper into the contemplative elements. It's a technique that works for your body and mind in all phases of life and is still relevant today.

III. Spreading the Knowledge: Motivating Others

Consider how Chair Yoga has improved your life and provided you joy. Think about imparting this knowledge to your friends, relatives, and neighbors. Organize Chair Yoga classes, talk about your experiences, and encourage people to start their own 30-day challenge. Well-being has far-reaching effects that go beyond individual practices.

As we come to the end of this comprehensive guide to 5-minute workouts, keep in mind that Chair Yoga is more than simply a physical regimen; it's a philosophy—a comprehensive approach to wellbeing that goes beyond the tangible. Let Chair Yoga become a sustaining practice and a lifelong partner on your path to inner peace, health, and vigor as you carry the lessons and advantages forward.